CARB CYCLING FOR WOMEN OVER 50

A Beginner's Ultimate Guide and cookbook to Weight Loss, Nutritious Meal Plans, and Simple Prep Recipes for over 50 and 60 "

Amos jimmy

Copyright © [2024] by [Amos jimmy]

All rights reserved. No part of this publication may be reproduced, distributed, or transmitted in any form or by any means, including photocopying, recording, or other electronic or mechanical methods, without the prior written permission of the publisher, except in the case of brief quotations embodied in critical reviews and certain other noncommercial uses permitted by copyright law.

TABLE OF CONTENT

CHAPTER 1 11
OVERVIEW OF CARB CYCLING 11
   How Does Carb Cycling Work? 12
   The Benefits for Women Over 50 and 60 13
   Understanding Carbohydrates and Their Role in the Body 15
   The Science Behind Carb Cycling and Weight Loss 16
   High-Carb Days: Purpose and Planning 18
      When to Schedule High-Carb Days 18
   Low-Carb Days: Purpose and Planning 19
      When to Schedule Low-Carb Days 19
      Low-Carb Day Planning 20

CHAPTER 2 21
HIGH CARBS BREAKFAST RECIPES 21
   Oatmeal with Mixed Berries and Nuts 21
   Quinoa Fruit Salad 24
   Sweet Potato and Black Bean Breakfast Burrito 26
   Banana Pancakes with Maple Syrup and Fresh Fruit 29
   Tropical Mango and Coconut Rice Pudding 32
LOW CARB BREAKFAST RECIPES 35

Avocado and Egg Breakfast Bowl 35

Smoked Salmon and Cream Cheese Roll-Ups 38

Mushroom and Spinach Frittata 40

Zucchini and Bell Pepper Mini Quiches 43

Cauliflower Hash Browns with Smoked Salmon 46

CHAPTER 3 51

HIGH CARB LUNCH RECIPES 51

Sweet Potato Chickpea Salad 51

Brown Rice Stir-Fry with Vegetables and Tofu 54

Pasta Primavera with Whole Wheat Pasta 56

Mediterranean Quinoa Salad 59

Sweet Potato Black Bean Burritos 62

LOW CARB LUNCH RECIPES 65

Grilled Chicken and Avocado Salad 65

Salmon and Asparagus Bundles 68

Beef and Broccoli Stir-Fry 71

Turkey Lettuce Wraps 73

Shrimp and Spinach Salad 76

CHAPTER 4 81

HIGH CARB SNACKS AND APPETIZER 81

Fruit and Oat Energy Balls 81

Sweet Potato Hummus with Whole Wheat Pita 84

High Carb Quinoa Fruit Salad 87

Baked Sweet Potato Fries with Greek Yogurt Dip 89

Quinoa and Black Bean Stuffed Peppers 92

LOW CARB SNACKS AND APPETIZER 95

Avocado Cucumber Rolls 95

Stuffed Mini Bell Peppers 98

Zucchini Chips with Herbed Yogurt Dip 100

Cauliflower Hummus with Vegetable Sticks 103

Avocado and Salmon Salad Cups 106

CHAPTER 5 110

HIGH CARB DINNER RECIPES 110

Gnocchi with Tomato Sauce and Fresh Basil 110

Seafood Alfredo Pasta 112

Eggplant Parmesan with Spaghetti 114

Korean BBQ Beef with Steamed Rice 116

Chicken Tikka Masala with Basmati Rice 118

LOW CARB DINNER RECIPES 121

Grilled Lemon-Herb Chicken and Zucchini 121

Beef and Mushroom Lettuce Wraps 124

Salmon and Avocado Salad 127

Herb-Crusted Pork Tenderloin with Roasted Asparagus 130

Grilled Chicken Caesar Salad 133

CHAPTER 6 136

7 DAYS DAILY MEAL PLAN 136

Monday: High-Carb + Strength Training 136

6:30 AM: Breakfast 136

9:00 AM: Workout 136

11:00 AM: Snack 136

1:00 PM: Lunch 136

4:00 PM: Snack 136

7:00 PM: Dinner 136

Tuesday: Low-Carb + Light Activity (Yoga or Walk) 137

7:00 AM: Breakfast 137

10:00 AM: Light Activity 137

12:00 PM: Lunch 137

3:00 PM: Snack 137

6:00 PM: Dinner 137

Wednesday: High-Carb + HIIT 137

6:30 AM: Breakfast 137

    9:00 AM: Workou 137

    11:00 AM: Snack 137

    1:00 PM: Lunch 137

    4:00 PM: Snack 138

    7:00 PM: Dinner 138

Thursday: Low-Carb + Rest Day 138

    7:00 AM: Breakfast 138

    Rest Day: 138

    12:00 PM: Lunch 138

    3:00 PM: Snack 138

    6:00 PM: Dinner 138

Friday: High-Carb + Circuit Training 138

    6:30 AM: Breakfast 138

    9:00 AM: Workout 138

    11:00 AM: Snack 138

    1:00 PM: Lunch 138

    4:00 PM: Snack 139

    7:00 PM: Dinner 139

Saturday: Low-Carb + Light Activity (Swimming or Cycling) 139

- 7:00 AM: Breakfast 139
- 10:00 AM: Light Activity 139
- 12:00 PM: Lunch 139
- 3:00 PM: Snack 139
- 6:00 PM: Dinner 139

Sunday: Low-Carb + Rest Day 139
- 8:00 AM: Breakfast 139
- Rest Day: 139
- 12:00 PM: 139
- 3:00 PM: Snack 140
- 6:00 PM: Dinner 140

2 WEEKS MEAL PLANNER 141
Jimmy Asking For An Honest Review 143

INTRODUCTION

Embarking on a journey to rediscover health and vitality in the golden years, "Carb Cycling for Women Over 50 and 60 Beyond" serves as a beacon of hope and transformation. In a world where nutrition advice often feels one-size-fits-all, this book carves out a much-needed space for women who stand at the intersection of wisdom and change. With a focus on carb cycling, a method that champions flexibility and balance, we aim to empower you to navigate the unique nutritional needs and challenges that arise with age.

This guide is more than just about losing weight; it's about cultivating a lifestyle that enhances your overall well-being, energy levels, and longevity. Whether you're looking to rejuvenate your metabolism, manage hormonal shifts, or simply embrace a healthier version of yourself, our approach is tailored to align with the changes your body undergoes past the age of 50.

Through a blend of science-backed insights and practical advice, we will walk you through the principles of carb cycling, how it can be adapted to suit your individual health goals, and the profound impact it can have on your life. Our mission is to provide you with the tools and knowledge to make informed choices about your diet, breaking down the complexities of nutrition into actionable steps that fit seamlessly into your life.

Join us on this transformative journey, where age is but a number, and the best years are yet to come. Together, we'll explore how the strategic inclusion and timing of carbohydrates can unlock a vibrant, healthier future, proving that it's never too late to turn a new leaf in the book of life.

CHAPTER 1

OVERVIEW OF CARB CYCLING

Carb cycling, a term that often circles the fitness and nutrition world with an aura of both curiosity and intrigue, stands as a unique approach to dieting that might just be the game changer for women over 50 and 60 looking to rejuvenate their health, boost their metabolism, and find a sustainable way to manage weight. Let's dive deep into this topic, in a way that feels like we're sharing a warm, friendly chat over a cup of tea.

At its core, carb cycling is a dietary approach that involves alternating between high-carb days and low-carb days. This isn't a one-size-fits-all kind of deal; rather, it's tailored to fit the individual's lifestyle, workout routine, and health goals. The concept behind it is pretty straightforward yet scientifically savvy. It's about manipulating your carbohydrate intake to fuel your body efficiently for workouts and recovery, while also optimizing fat loss and muscle gain. But, why does this matter more for women over 50?

As we age, our bodies undergo various changes. For women crossing the milestone of 50, these changes become more pronounced due to menopause. Reduced estrogen levels can affect metabolism, making it easier to gain weight, especially around the abdomen. Moreover, the risk of developing conditions like type 2 diabetes and cardiovascular diseases also increases. Muscle mass naturally declines with age, slowing down the metabolic rate. Here's where carb cycling can step in as a knight in shining armor.

How Does Carb Cycling Work?

Carb cycling targets these issues by alternating carbohydrate intake, which can help manage blood sugar levels, support weight management, and even encourage muscle maintenance and growth when paired with resistance training. On high-carb days, when you're likely to engage in more intense workouts, your body gets the energy it needs for those activities and for recovery afterward. Low-carb days help with fat burning and insulin sensitivity, as your body is encouraged to use fat for fuel instead of carbs.

The Benefits for Women Over 50 and 60

Now, let's talk about the real meat of the matter—the benefits of carb cycling specifically for women over 50 and 60.

- **Improved Metabolic Flexibility**: As we age, our metabolic flexibility—our body's ability to switch between burning carbs and fats for energy—can decrease. Carb cycling helps improve this flexibility, making it easier for the body to adapt to different energy sources, which can be beneficial for weight management and overall energy levels.
- **Weight Management**: By optimizing when and how carbs are consumed, carb cycling can aid in weight loss or maintenance. This is particularly important for postmenopausal women, who might find that their usual diets don't work as effectively as they used to for managing weight.
- **Supports Muscle Mass**: Maintaining muscle mass is crucial as we age, not just for metabolism but also for bone health, balance, and overall strength. High-carb days support muscle growth and repair, especially if they're timed with resistance training sessions.

- **Hormonal Balance:** The fluctuations in carb intake can also have a positive effect on hormones, particularly insulin, which helps regulate blood sugar levels. For women over 50, who might be more prone to insulin resistance, this can be a significant benefit.
- **Flexibility and Sustainability**: Unlike strict low-carb or ketogenic diets, carb cycling offers a more flexible approach that can be more sustainable in the long run. It allows for social meals and treats, making it easier to stick to and integrate into a healthy lifestyle.

Understanding Carbohydrates and Their Role in the Body

we're embarking on this journey to understand carbs better. You've probably heard all sorts of things about carbohydrates, right? Some people villainize them, while others can't seem to get enough. But what's the real deal with carbs, especially for us, ladies over 50?

First off, carbohydrates are one of the three macronutrients, alongside proteins and fats, that our bodies need to function properly. They're our primary energy source, kind of like fuel for a car. When you eat carbs, your body breaks them down into glucose, which is then used to power everything from your brain to your muscles. Pretty important, right?

But here's where it gets interesting. Not all carbs are created equal. We have simple carbohydrates, found in sugary snacks and processed foods, which can spike our blood sugar levels quickly.

Then, there are complex carbohydrates, found in whole grains, vegetables, and legumes, which are digested more slowly and provide a more steady energy source. For us, especially as we navigate the changes in our bodies post-50, opting for complex carbs is the way to go. They help keep our energy levels stable, support our digestion, and can even help manage weight.

The Science Behind Carb Cycling and Weight Loss

Like we said before now. Carb cycling involves varying your carbohydrate intake on a daily or weekly basis. Some days you'll eat more carbs, and some days you'll eat less. Why do this, you ask? Well, it's all about working with your body's metabolism to potentially aid in weight loss or management, and improve overall health.

As women over 50, our bodies go through significant changes, including shifts in hormone levels that can affect our metabolism and how we store fat. It's no secret that losing weight can become a bit more challenging at this stage of life. That's where carb cycling can come in handy. By alternating between high-carb and low-carb days, you can potentially trick your body into burning fat more efficiently, rather than relying on glucose (from carbs) for energy.

On high-carb days, you're essentially refueling your body's energy stores, which is great for those days when you're more active or hitting the gym. Think of it as giving your metabolism a little boost. On low-carb days, your body, in the absence of its primary energy source (glucose), starts to look for other sources of fuel, namely fat. This process can help with weight loss and can also be beneficial for blood sugar management, which is super important as we get older.

It's crucial, though, to approach carb cycling in a healthy, balanced way. This isn't about cutting out carbs entirely or going to extremes. It's about smartly varying your carb intake to work with your body's natural rhythms and needs. And remember, the quality of the carbs matters a lot. On your high-carb days, you still want to focus on those nutrient-rich, complex carbohydrates that will nourish your body and support your health goals.

High-Carb Days: Purpose and Planning

High-carb days are not just about indulging in your favorite carb-rich foods; they have a specific purpose in your nutrition strategy. These days are designed to replenish your glycogen stores, which is the stored form of energy in your muscles and liver. Replenishing glycogen is crucial for maintaining energy levels, supporting recovery after workouts, and ensuring your metabolism functions efficiently.

When to Schedule High-Carb Days

Planning high-carb days strategically throughout your week can maximize their benefits. A common approach is to align high-carb days with your most intense workout days. For instance, if you're focusing on strength training or endurance activities, scheduling high-carb days on or around these sessions can enhance performance, support muscle recovery, and maintain energy levels.

For women over 50 and 60, incorporating **2-3 high-carb days** per week is a good starting point. These days could be spaced out, **such as on Monday, Wednesday, and Friday, to coincide with workout days**, ensuring your body has the energy it needs to perform and recover.

High-Carb Day Planning

On high-carb days, focus on incorporating healthy carb sources like whole grains, fruits, vegetables, and legumes. These foods provide not only the necessary carbs but also fiber, vitamins, and minerals. Planning your meals around your workouts can also optimize nutrient uptake and use. For example, having a carb-rich meal 2-3 hours before your workout can ensure you have ample energy, while a similar meal post-workout can aid in recovery.

Low-Carb Days: Purpose and Planning

Low-carb days serve a different but equally important purpose. By reducing carbohydrate intake, you're encouraging your body to burn stored fat for energy, which can support weight loss and improve body composition. Low-carb days also help regulate blood sugar levels and can improve insulin sensitivity, which is particularly beneficial for women over 50 and 60, who may be experiencing changes in how their bodies manage blood sugar.

When to Schedule Low-Carb Days
Scheduling low-carb days is as important as planning high-carb days. These days are typically aligned with lighter workout days or rest days since your body's demand for glycogen is lower. For a balanced approach, you might

alternate high-carb and low-carb days throughout the week or follow a pattern that suits your lifestyle and fitness schedule best.

An example schedule could involve high-carb days on **Monday, Wednesday, and Friday**, with low-carb days on **Tuesday, Thursday, Saturday, and Sunday**. This pattern ensures that your body receives the energy it needs on workout days while still promoting fat burning and insulin sensitivity on rest days.

Low-Carb Day Planning
On low-carb days, prioritize high-quality protein sources, healthy fats, and low-carb vegetables. These nutrients will support muscle maintenance, provide lasting energy, and keep you feeling full. Foods like lean meats, fish, eggs, nuts, seeds, and leafy greens should be staples on low-carb days.

Planning meals that are satisfying and nutritious can help prevent cravings and make low-carb days enjoyable rather than a chore. Incorporating variety, such as different protein sources and vegetables, can keep meals interesting and ensure you're getting a range of nutrients. Now we will look at the ingredient

CHAPTER 2

HIGH CARBS BREAKFAST RECIPES

Oatmeal with Mixed Berries and Nuts

Serves: 1

Cooking Time: 15 minutes

Ingredients:

- Rolled oats (high carb friendly): 1 cup
- Almond milk or water (for those intolerant to dairy): 2 cups
- Mixed berries (blueberries, strawberries, raspberries - high in antioxidants): 1/2 cup
- Chia seeds (fiber and omega-3 fatty acids): 2 tablespoons
- Walnuts or almonds, chopped (healthy fats and proteins; for nut allergies, substitute with sunflower seeds): 1/4 cup
- Honey or maple syrup (natural sweetener, optional): 1 tablespoon

Instructions:

- In a medium saucepan, bring the almond milk (or water) to a boil. Add the rolled oats and reduce the heat to medium. Stir occasionally and cook for about 5 minutes.
- While the oats are cooking, chop the walnuts or almonds (or prepare the sunflower seeds if using them as a substitute) and set them aside.
- Once the oats are cooked and have absorbed most of the liquid, remove the saucepan from heat. Stir in the mixed berries, chia seeds, and chopped nuts. Allow the mixture to sit for a couple of minutes; the heat will slightly soften the berries and nuts.
- Serve the oatmeal in a bowl. If desired, drizzle honey or maple syrup on top for added sweetness.

Note: Benefits of the Recipe

- Rolled oats are a great source of complex carbohydrates, providing sustained energy. They also contain beta-glucan, a type of soluble fiber that has been shown to improve cholesterol levels and heart health.

- Berries are low in calories but high in fiber, vitamins, and antioxidants, which are crucial for reducing inflammation and protecting heart health.
- Nuts and seeds provide healthy fats, proteins, and fiber, supporting heart health and satiety. Chia seeds, in particular, are rich in omega-3 fatty acids, which are beneficial for brain health.

Nutritional Information (approximation):

- Calories: 500 kcal
- Carbohydrates: 75 g
- Fiber: 15 g
- Sugars: 20 g (includes natural sugars from fruits and optional sweetener)
- Protein: 15 g
- Fat: 20 g
- Saturated Fat: 2 g
- Cholesterol: 0 mg
- Sodium: 30 mg (varies with the addition of salt or use of sweeteners)

Quinoa Fruit Salad

Serves: 1

Cooking Time: 0 minutes (assuming quinoa is precooked)

Ingredients:

- Quinoa (high carb, high protein): 1 cup cooked
- Diced apple (fiber and vitamins; for those with fructose intolerance, substitute with orange segments): 1 medium
- Sliced strawberries (high in antioxidants): 1/2 cup
- Blueberries (antioxidants and vitamins): 1/2 cup
- Greek yogurt or coconut yogurt (for dairy intolerance): 1/2 cup
- Honey or maple syrup (optional): 1 tablespoon
- Cinnamon (antioxidant properties): 1/2 teaspoon

Instructions:

- In a large bowl, mix the cooked quinoa with the diced apple, sliced strawberries, and blueberries.
- Add the Greek yogurt (or coconut yogurt) to the bowl. Drizzle the honey or maple syrup over the top and sprinkle with cinnamon.

- Gently mix all the ingredients until they are well combined.
- Serve immediately, or refrigerate for a chilled salad.

Note: Benefits of the Recipe

- Quinoa is a complete protein, providing all nine essential amino acids, and is high in fiber and iron, making it an excellent choice for a high-carb breakfast.
- Fresh fruit provides natural sugars for energy, along with dietary fiber, vitamins, and antioxidants that support overall health and well-being.
- Greek yogurt adds protein and probiotics, which are beneficial for gut health. For those intolerant to dairy, coconut yogurt is a lactose-free alternative that also offers probiotics.

Nutritional Information (approximation):

- Calories: 450 kcal
- Carbohydrates: 85 g
- Fiber: 10 g
- Sugars: 30 g (includes natural sugars from fruits and optional sweetener)
- Protein: 15 g

- Fat: 5 g
- Sodium: 50 mg

Sweet Potato and Black Bean Breakfast Burrito

Serves: 2

Cooking Time: 25 minutes (for roasting sweet potatoes)

Ingredients:

- Sweet potatoes (high carb, rich in vitamins A and C): 1 large, cubed and roasted
- Black beans (fiber and protein; for those with legume intolerance, substitute with scrambled tofu): 1 cup
- Whole wheat or corn tortilla (for gluten intolerance, choose gluten-free tortillas): 2 large
- Avocado (healthy fats and fiber): 1/2, sliced
- Salsa (flavor and minimal calories): to taste
- Spinach leaves (vitamins, minerals, and fiber): 1/2 cup

Instructions:

- Preheat the oven to 400°F (200°C). Toss the cubed sweet potatoes in a little olive oil and spread them on a baking sheet. Roast in the oven for about 20-25 minutes or until tender.
- Warm the black beans (and scramble the tofu if using as a substitute) in a pan over medium heat.
- Warm the tortillas on a skillet for about 30 seconds on each side.
- Assemble the burritos by laying down the tortillas and adding an even layer of roasted sweet potatoes, black beans (or scrambled tofu), sliced avocado, salsa, and spinach leaves.
- Roll up the tortillas, folding in the sides to enclose the filling.
- Serve immediately or wrap in foil to keep warm.

Note: Benefits of the Recipe

- Sweet potatoes are a nutritious source of carbohydrates, rich in beta-carotene, vitamins A and C, and fiber, which support immune function and gut health.

- Black beans provide plant-based protein and fiber, which can help regulate blood sugar levels and are beneficial for heart health.
- Whole grains, like those in whole wheat tortillas, are linked to a lower risk of heart disease, diabetes, and certain cancers. They provide necessary fiber for digestion and long-lasting energy.

Nutritional Information (approximation per serving):

- Calories: 600 kcal
- Carbohydrates: 90 g
- Fiber: 15 g
- Sugars: 8 g
- Protein: 20 g
- Fat: 20 g
- Sodium: 400 mg

Banana Pancakes with Maple Syrup and Fresh Fruit

Serves: 2

Cooking Time: 15 minutes

Ingredients:

- Whole wheat flour (high carb, high fiber; for gluten intolerance, substitute with oat flour): 1 cup
- Ripe bananas (natural sweetness and high carbs): 2 medium, mashed
- Almond milk or any plant-based milk (for those intolerant to dairy): 1 cup
- Baking powder: 2 teaspoons
- Egg (protein; for egg allergies, substitute with flaxseed meal mixed with water): 1 large
- Maple syrup (natural sweetener): to serve
- Fresh fruit (antioxidants, vitamins): 1/2 cup (berries, sliced banana, or apple)

Instructions:

- In a large mixing bowl, combine the whole wheat (or oat) flour and baking powder.

- In another bowl, mix the mashed bananas, plant-based milk, and egg (or flaxseed meal mixture).
- Pour the wet ingredients into the dry ingredients and stir until just combined. Avoid overmixing to keep the pancakes fluffy.
- Heat a non-stick skillet over medium heat. Pour 1/4 cup of batter for each pancake and cook until bubbles form on the surface, then flip and cook until golden brown.
- Serve the pancakes warm, topped with maple syrup and fresh fruit.

Note: Benefits of the Recipe

- Whole wheat flour is a good source of complex carbohydrates and dietary fiber, which helps in maintaining stable blood sugar levels and promoting satiety.
- Bananas provide a quick source of energy through their high carbohydrate content and also supply potassium, which is vital for muscle and nerve function.
- Plant-based milks are often fortified with calcium and vitamin D, essential for bone health, especially important for individuals over 50 and 60.

- The use of fresh fruit adds additional fiber, vitamins, and antioxidants, aiding in digestion and providing essential nutrients for overall health.

Nutritional Information (approximation per serving):

- Calories: 400 kcal
- Carbohydrates: 80 g
- Fiber: 10 g
- Sugars: 20 g (natural sugars from bananas and optional sweetener)
- Protein: 10 g
- Fat: 5 g
- Cholesterol: 93 mg (if using eggs)
- Sodium: 300 mg

Tropical Mango and Coconut Rice Pudding

Serves: 4

Cooking Time: 45 minutes

Ingredients:

- Jasmine rice or short-grain rice (high carb; for a more exotic twist, use black rice, which is also high in antioxidants): 1 cup
- Coconut milk (for lactose intolerance, already suitable; rich in medium-chain triglycerides (MCTs)): 2 cups
- Mango, diced (high in dietary fiber, vitamins A and C): 1 large
- Honey or maple syrup (optional sweetener): 2 tablespoons
- Chia seeds (fiber and omega-3s; for those with difficulty digesting seeds, omit or blend into the mixture for easier digestion): 1 tablespoon
- A pinch of salt (enhances flavor)

Instructions:

- In a medium saucepan, bring the coconut milk to a simmer. Add the rice and a pinch of salt, then reduce the heat to low.
- Cover and cook for 20-25 minutes, or until the rice is tender and the mixture has thickened. Stir occasionally to prevent sticking.
- Once the rice is cooked, remove from heat and let it cool slightly. Stir in the honey or maple syrup, chia seeds, and half of the diced mango.
- Serve the rice pudding in bowls, topped with the remaining diced mango.

Note: Benefits of the Recipe

- Rice is a fundamental high-carbohydrate food that provides a significant energy source for high carb days. It also serves as a good base for various nutrients when paired with fruits and seeds.
- Coconut milk not only adds a creamy texture and flavor but also provides a source of healthy fats, particularly medium-chain triglycerides, which are processed differently by the body, potentially aiding in energy expenditure and weight management.
- Mangoes are not only sweet and satisfying but also packed with vitamins A and C, promoting skin health

and immune function. Their high fiber content can aid in digestion and help prevent constipation.
- Chia seeds are a superfood providing omega-3 fatty acids, important for heart health and cognitive function, along with fiber for digestive health.

Nutritional Information (approximation per serving):

- Calories: 350 kcal
- Carbohydrates: 60 g
- Fiber: 5 g
- Sugars: 15 g (includes natural sugars from mango and optional sweetener)
- Protein: 5 g
- Fat: 10 g
- Saturated Fat: 8 g (from coconut milk)
- Cholesterol: 0 mg
- Sodium: 50 mg

LOW CARB BREAKFAST RECIPES

Avocado and Egg Breakfast Bowl

Serves: 1

Cooking Time: 15 minutes

Ingredients:

- 1 medium avocado, sliced (healthy fats, low carb)
- 2 large eggs (protein; for those with egg allergies, substitute with silken tofu scrambled with turmeric)
- 2 cups spinach (low carb, high in iron and vitamins)
- 1/2 cup cherry tomatoes, halved (low carb, high in antioxidants; for nightshade intolerance, omit or substitute with sliced cucumber)
- 1 tablespoon olive oil (healthy fats)
- Salt and pepper, to taste

Instructions:

- Heat the olive oil in a non-stick skillet over medium heat. Crack the eggs into the skillet and fry to your preference, seasoning with salt and pepper. Alternatively, if using silken tofu, scramble it in the

skillet with a pinch of turmeric, salt, and pepper until heated through.
- While the eggs are cooking, wash the spinach and cherry tomatoes. If using cucumber, slice it now.
- On a serving bowl or plate, arrange the sliced avocado, cooked eggs or scrambled tofu, spinach, and cherry tomatoes or cucumber slices.
- Season the entire bowl with a pinch of salt and pepper to taste. Serve immediately.
- Note: Benefits of the Recipe

- Avocados are rich in monounsaturated fats, which can help reduce LDL cholesterol levels and are beneficial for heart health.
- Eggs provide a high-quality protein source, essential for muscle maintenance and repair, and are rich in vitamins D and B12, important for bone health and energy metabolism, respectively.
- Spinach is a nutrient-dense vegetable, high in iron, which is crucial for preventing anemia, a common issue in older women.

Nutritional Information (per serving):

- Calories: Approximately 450 kcal
- Protein: 15 g
- Total Fat: 35 g
- Saturated Fat: 6 g
- Monounsaturated Fat: 15 g
- Carbohydrates: 18 g
- Dietary Fiber: 10 g
- Sugars: 4 g

Smoked Salmon and Cream Cheese Roll-Ups

Serves: 2

Cooking Time: 10 minutes

Ingredients:

- 4 ounces smoked salmon (protein and omega-3 fatty acids; for those who avoid fish, substitute with thinly sliced tofu or tempeh)
- 2 tablespoons cream cheese (fat; for dairy intolerance, use dairy-free cream cheese alternatives)
- 1 small cucumber, sliced thinly (hydration and vitamins)
- 1 teaspoon capers (optional, for added flavor)
- Dill, to taste (optional, for flavor)
- A squeeze of lemon juice (vitamin C, to taste)

Instructions:

- Lay out the slices of smoked salmon on a flat surface. If using a substitute like tofu or tempeh, ensure they are thinly sliced and patted dry.
- Spread a thin layer of cream cheese or dairy-free alternative evenly over each salmon slice.

- Arrange the thinly sliced cucumber over the cream cheese. Sprinkle capers and dill across the cucumber, if using.
- Carefully roll up the salmon slices into tight rolls. Secure with a toothpick if necessary.
- Just before serving, drizzle a bit of lemon juice over the roll-ups for a fresh, citrusy accent.

Note: Benefits of the Recipe

- Smoked salmon is an excellent source of omega-3 fatty acids, essential for maintaining heart health and reducing inflammation.
- Cream cheese can be replaced with dairy-free alternatives, catering to those with dairy intolerances, ensuring the meal remains low in carbs.
- Cucumbers are a hydrating vegetable, adding volume to meals without significant calories or carbs, and providing essential vitamins.

Nutritional Information (per serving):

- Calories: Approximately 200 kcal
- Protein: 15 g
- Total Fat: 14 g
- Saturated Fat: 6 g

- Carbohydrates: 3 g
- Dietary Fiber: 0.5 g
- Sugars: 2 g
- Cholesterol: 50 mg (if using dairy cream cheese)

Mushroom and Spinach Frittata

Serves: 4

Cooking Time: 25 minutes

Ingredients:

- 6 large eggs (high-quality protein; for allergies, use chickpea flour mixed with water to form a batter)
- 1 cup mushrooms, sliced (low carb, rich in selenium and vitamin D)
- 2 cups spinach (iron and vitamins)
- 1/4 cup crumbled feta cheese (for dairy intolerance, substitute with nutritional yeast for a cheesy flavor without the dairy)
- 1 tablespoon olive oil (healthy fats)
- Salt and pepper, to taste

Instructions:

- Preheat your oven to 375°F (190°C).
- In a large mixing bowl, beat the eggs (or prepare the chickpea batter) with salt and pepper.
- Heat the olive oil in a 10-inch ovenproof skillet over medium heat. Add the mushrooms and sauté until they're soft, about 5 minutes.
- Add the spinach to the skillet and cook until wilted, about 2 minutes.
- Pour the beaten eggs or chickpea batter over the vegetables in the skillet, stirring gently to ensure an even distribution.
- Sprinkle the crumbled feta cheese or nutritional yeast evenly over the top.
- Transfer the skillet to the oven and bake until the frittata is set and golden on top, about 15 minutes.
- Let cool for a few minutes before slicing and serving.

Note: Benefits of the Recipe

- Mushrooms are one of the few non-animal sources of vitamin D, essential for bone health.

- The combination of eggs (or chickpea flour) and vegetables ensures a high intake of proteins and vitamins while keeping the carb content low.
- Feta cheese adds calcium for bone health, but nutritional yeast is a great dairy-free alternative, providing B vitamins.

Nutritional Information (per serving):

- Calories: Approximately 220 kcal
- Protein: 18 g
- Total Fat: 15 g
- Saturated Fat: 5 g
- Carbohydrates: 5 g
- Dietary Fiber: 1 g
- Sugars: 2 g
- Cholesterol: 280 mg (if using eggs)

Zucchini and Bell Pepper Mini Quiches

Serves: 12 mini quiches

Cooking Time: 30 minutes

Ingredients:

- 1 cup grated zucchini (low carb, high in fiber)
- 1/2 cup diced bell peppers (low carb, high in vitamins A and C; for nightshade intolerance, substitute with diced asparagus)
- 6 large eggs (high in protein and vitamins D, B6, and B12; for egg allergies, substitute with a mixture of chickpea flour and water)
- 1/2 cup shredded cheddar cheese (for dairy intolerance, use dairy-free cheese)
- 1 tablespoon coconut oil (for greasing muffin tins)
- Salt and pepper, to taste

Instructions:

- Preheat your oven to 375°F (190°C). Use the coconut oil to grease a 12-cup muffin tin.
- In a large bowl, beat the eggs (or prepare the chickpea flour mixture) and season with salt and pepper.

- Squeeze any excess moisture from the grated zucchini using a clean kitchen towel or paper towels.
- Add the grated zucchini, diced bell peppers (or asparagus), and shredded cheese to the egg mixture. Stir to combine.
- Pour the mixture evenly into the greased muffin cups, filling each about two-thirds full.
- Bake in the preheated oven until the mini quiches are set and lightly golden on top, about 20-25 minutes.
- Allow to cool for a few minutes before removing from the muffin tin. Serve warm.

Note: Benefits of the Recipe

- Zucchini is low in carbs and contains vitamins B6, riboflavin, and manganese, essential for energy production and overall health.
- Bell peppers are a rich source of antioxidants, particularly vitamin C, which supports immune function and skin health.
- Eggs provide a complete source of protein, essential for muscle maintenance and repair, and are also rich in selenium and choline, important for thyroid function and brain health.

Nutritional Information (per mini quiche):

- Calories: Approximately 100 kcal
- Protein: 7 g
- Total Fat: 7 g
- Saturated Fat: 3 g
- Carbohydrates: 2 g
- Dietary Fiber: 0.5 g
- Sugars: 1 g
- Cholesterol: 95 mg (if using eggs)

Cauliflower Hash Browns with Smoked Salmon

Serves: 4

Cooking Time: 20 minutes

Ingredients:

- 2 cups riced cauliflower (low carb, high in fiber, vitamins C, K, and B6; for those with cruciferous vegetable sensitivity, substitute with shredded turnips)
- 4 ounces smoked salmon (omega-3 fatty acids and protein; for vegetarians, substitute with avocado slices for healthy fats)
- 1 large egg (binds the hash browns together; for egg allergies, substitute with ground flaxseed mixed with water)
- 1/4 cup chopped green onions (for flavor; for those sensitive to alliums, omit or use chives)
- 2 tablespoons olive oil (for frying)
- Salt and pepper, to taste

Instructions:

- In a large bowl, combine the riced cauliflower, chopped green onions, and salt and pepper. Mix well.
- Beat the egg (or prepare the flaxseed mixture) and add it to the cauliflower mixture, stirring until evenly combined.
- Heat the olive oil in a large skillet over medium heat. Scoop portions of the cauliflower mixture into the skillet, pressing down to form patties.
- Cook the hash browns until golden and crispy on both sides, about 3-4 minutes per side.
- Serve the hash browns topped with smoked salmon (or avocado slices for a vegetarian option).

Note: Benefits of the Recipe

- Cauliflower provides a low-carb alternative to traditional hash browns, offering fiber, vitamins C, K, and B6 for digestive health, immune function, and bone health.
- Smoked salmon offers omega-3 fatty acids, essential for heart health and cognitive function, making it particularly important for women over 50 and 60.

- Olive oil contributes monounsaturated fats and antioxidants, supporting heart health and providing anti-inflammatory benefits.

Nutritional Information (per serving):

- Calories: Approximately 220 kcal
- Protein: 14 g
- Total Fat: 15 g
- Saturated Fat: 3 g
- Carbohydrates: 8 g
- Dietary Fiber: 3 g
- Sugars: 3 g
- Cholesterol: 60 mg (if using eggs)

CONGRATULATIONS ON COMPLETING CHAPTER 2 OF OUR CARB CYCLING GUIDE

We sincerely hope that the breakfast recipes for high carb and low carb provided have not only tantalized your taste buds but also supported you in your journey towards managing carb intake effectively.

Each recipe within our guide has been meticulously designed to align with carb cycling principles, ensuring that you can enjoy your meals without concern for disrupting your dietary goals. Embracing these recipes signifies a proactive step in enhancing your overall health and well-being.

As we eagerly anticipate introducing you to an array of lunch options in Chapter 3, we pause to seek your valued feedback.

Your insights and honest review of the breakfast recipes are crucial for us. They enable us to refine our approach, ensuring that we meet your expectations and assist others in navigating their carb cycling journey with greater confidence.

Thank you for contributing to our community's growth and for your commitment to exploring the carb cycling lifestyle. We are excited to guide you through the forthcoming chapter, where delicious, carb-conscious lunch recipes await.

Your involvement is key to our collective success, and we look forward to hearing from you.

CHAPTER 3

HIGH CARB LUNCH RECIPES

Sweet Potato Chickpea Salad

Serves: 4

Cooking Time: 30 minutes

Ingredients:

- 2 cups cubed sweet potatoes (high in complex carbs and fiber; for beta-carotene sensitivity, substitute with butternut squash)
- 1 cup cooked chickpeas (high carb, high fiber; for legume intolerance, substitute with quinoa)
- 1 cup cooked quinoa (high carb, high protein)
- 2 cups spinach leaves (nutrient-dense, low carb)
- 1/4 cup thinly sliced red onion (flavor; for those sensitive to alliums, substitute with sliced bell peppers)
- 3 tablespoons olive oil (for roasting sweet potatoes and dressing)
- 2 tablespoons lemon juice (vitamin C)
- Salt and pepper, to taste

Instructions:

- Preheat the oven to 400°F (200°C). Toss the cubed sweet potatoes with 1 tablespoon of olive oil, salt, and pepper. Spread them on a baking sheet and roast until tender and slightly caramelized, about 20-25 minutes.
- In a large bowl, combine the cooked quinoa, cooked chickpeas, spinach leaves, and sliced red onion (or bell pepper).
- Once the sweet potatoes are roasted, add them to the bowl with the salad mixture.
- Whisk together the remaining 2 tablespoons of olive oil and lemon juice for the dressing. Season with salt and pepper to taste.
- Pour the dressing over the salad and toss gently to combine all the ingredients.
- Serve the salad warm or at room temperature.

Note: Benefits of the Recipe

- Sweet potatoes are a rich source of complex carbohydrates and dietary fiber, contributing to stable blood sugar levels and eye health.
- Chickpeas and quinoa provide a good balance of carbohydrates and protein, supporting energy levels and muscle maintenance.

- Spinach adds a nutrient-dense element, offering vitamins and minerals essential for overall health.

Nutritional Information (per serving):

- Calories: Approximately 350 kcal
- Protein: 10 g
- Total Fat: 10 g
- Saturated Fat: 1.5 g
- Carbohydrates: 55 g
- Dietary Fiber: 10 g
- Sugars: 5 g
- Sodium: 200 mg (varies with salt and dressing)

Brown Rice Stir-Fry with Vegetables and Tofu

Serves: 4

Cooking Time: 20 minutes

Ingredients:

- 2 cups cooked brown rice (high carb, rich in fiber; for intolerance, substitute with cauliflower rice)
- 1 cup cubed firm tofu (high in protein; for soy allergies, substitute with chickpea tempeh)
- 1 cup chopped broccoli (fiber, vitamins C and K; for sensitivity, substitute with zucchini)
- 1/2 cup sliced carrots (high in beta-carotene)
- 1/2 cup sliced bell peppers (vitamin C and antioxidants)
- 2 tablespoons soy sauce (umami flavor; for soy intolerance, use coconut aminos)
- 1 tablespoon sesame oil (healthy fats)
- 2 cloves minced garlic (antimicrobial properties; for intolerance, omit or use a pinch of asafoetida)
- Salt and pepper, to taste

Instructions:

- Heat the sesame oil in a large skillet or wok over medium-high heat.
- Add the garlic (or asafoetida), tofu, and vegetables to the skillet. Stir-fry for about 5-7 minutes, or until the vegetables are tender and the tofu is golden brown.
- Stir in the cooked brown rice and soy sauce (or coconut aminos). Cook for another 3-5 minutes, stirring frequently, until everything is heated through and well combined.
- Season with salt and pepper to taste. Serve hot.

Note: Benefits of the Recipe

- Brown rice provides sustained energy through complex carbohydrates and is rich in selenium for thyroid health.
- Tofu and vegetables contribute protein, calcium, iron, and essential vitamins, supporting bone health, anemia prevention, and antioxidant intake.

Nutritional Information (per serving):

- Calories: Approximately 300 kcal
- Protein: 12 g
- Total Fat: 7 g

- Saturated Fat: 1 g
- Carbohydrates: 50 g
- Dietary Fiber: 6 g
- Sugars: 3 g
- Sodium: 600 mg (varies with soy sauce and salt)

Pasta Primavera with Whole Wheat Pasta

Serves: 4

Cooking Time: 20 minutes

Ingredients:

- 2 cups cooked whole wheat pasta (high in complex carbs and fiber; for gluten intolerance, substitute with lentil or chickpea pasta)
- 2 cups chopped assorted vegetables (zucchini, asparagus, cherry tomatoes; high in vitamins and fiber)
- 2 tablespoons olive oil
- 2 cloves minced garlic (for intolerance, omit or substitute with chives)
- 1/4 cup grated Parmesan cheese (for dairy intolerance, substitute with nutritional yeast)
- 1/4 cup chopped fresh basil
- Salt and pepper, to taste

Instructions:

- Heat the olive oil in a large skillet over medium heat. Add the garlic (or chives) and sauté until fragrant, about 1 minute.
- Add the assorted vegetables to the skillet and cook until tender, about 5-7 minutes.
- Toss the cooked vegetables with the cooked whole wheat pasta, fresh basil, and grated Parmesan cheese (or nutritional yeast). Season with salt and pepper to taste.
- Serve warm, garnished with extra basil and cheese if desired.

Note: Benefits of the Recipe

- Whole wheat pasta offers a healthier, high-carb option with more nutrients and fiber compared to white pasta.
- The variety of vegetables increases dietary fiber and nutrient intake, supporting digestive health and reducing inflammation.
- Olive oil and Parmesan cheese (or nutritional yeast) add healthy fats and nutrients, including calcium and B vitamins, important for energy production and heart health.

Nutritional Information (per serving):

- Calories: Approximately 350 kcal
- Protein: 14 g
- Total Fat: 10 g
- Saturated Fat: 2 g
- Carbohydrates: 55 g
- Dietary Fiber: 8 g
- Sugars: 4 g
- Sodium: 200 mg (varies with Parmesan and salt)

Mediterranean Quinoa Salad

Serves: 4

Cooking Time: 15 minutes (excluding quinoa cooking time)

Ingredients:

- 1 cup cooked quinoa (high carb, complete protein; for quinoa sensitivity, substitute with couscous)
- 1/2 cup diced cucumber (hydration and vitamins; for cucumber intolerance, substitute with celery)
- 1/2 cup halved cherry tomatoes (vitamin C and potassium; for nightshade intolerance, use diced carrots)
- 1/4 cup sliced Kalamata olives (healthy fats)
- 1/4 cup crumbled feta cheese (calcium; for dairy intolerance, substitute with crumbled tofu)
- 1/4 cup finely chopped red onion (flavor; for those sensitive to alliums, omit or substitute with a sprinkle of paprika for color and mild flavor)
- 2 tablespoons olive oil (monounsaturated fats)
- 2 tablespoons lemon juice (vitamin C and flavor)
- 2 tablespoons chopped fresh parsley (vitamins A and C)

Instructions:

- In a large mixing bowl, combine the cooked quinoa, diced cucumber (or celery), halved cherry tomatoes (or diced carrots), sliced Kalamata olives, and crumbled feta cheese (or crumbled tofu).
- Add the finely chopped red onion (or sprinkle of paprika) to the bowl.
- In a small bowl, whisk together the olive oil and lemon juice. Pour this dressing over the salad mixture.
- Add the chopped fresh parsley to the salad and gently toss all the ingredients until well mixed.
- Season with salt and pepper to taste. Serve the salad chilled or at room temperature.

Note: Benefits of the Recipe

- Quinoa provides a complete source of protein and carbohydrates, ideal for energy and muscle repair.
- Olive oil contains monounsaturated fats, beneficial for heart health.
- Feta cheese offers calcium necessary for bone health, making it especially important for women over 50 and 60.

Nutritional Information (per serving):

- Calories: Approximately 250 kcal
- Protein: 8 g
- Total Fat: 14 g
- Saturated Fat: 3 g
- Carbohydrates: 24 g
- Dietary Fiber: 4 g
- Sugars: 3 g
- Sodium: 300 mg (varies with feta cheese and olives)

Sweet Potato Black Bean Burritos

Serves: 2

Cooking Time: 30 minutes

Ingredients:

- 1 cup cubed and roasted sweet potatoes (high in complex carbs and vitamin A; for sensitivity, use butternut squash)
- 1 cup cooked black beans (fiber and protein; for legume intolerance, substitute with roasted cauliflower)
- 2 large whole wheat tortillas (high carb; for gluten intolerance, use corn tortillas)
- 1 medium avocado, sliced (healthy fats and fiber)
- 1/2 cup raw spinach (iron and vitamins)
- 2 tablespoons salsa (flavor; for nightshade intolerance, use mashed avocado with lime)
- 1 teaspoon cumin (for flavor)
- 1 tablespoon lime juice (vitamin C and flavor)

Instructions:

- Preheat the oven to 350°F (175°C) if you prefer your burritos warmed.

- Lay out the whole wheat (or corn) tortillas on a flat surface.
- Divide the roasted sweet potatoes (or butternut squash), cooked black beans (or roasted cauliflower), sliced avocado, and raw spinach evenly among the tortillas.
- Add a tablespoon of salsa (or mashed avocado with lime) to each tortilla. Sprinkle with cumin and drizzle with lime juice.
- Carefully roll up the tortillas, folding in the sides to contain the filling.
- If desired, place the burritos in the oven for about 5-10 minutes to warm through.
- Serve the burritos hot, with extra salsa or avocado on the side if desired.

Note: Benefits of the Recipe

- Sweet potatoes are a rich source of carbohydrates and beta-carotene, important for vision, immune function, and skin health.
- Black beans provide fiber and protein, aiding in satiety and energy stability.

- Whole wheat tortillas contribute to the intake of nutrients and fiber, offering sustained energy and supporting digestive health.

Nutritional Information (per serving):

- Calories: Approximately 450 kcal
- Protein: 14 g
- Total Fat: 15 g
- Saturated Fat: 2.5 g
- Carbohydrates: 70 g
- Dietary Fiber: 15 g
- Sugars: 5 g
- Sodium: 500 mg (varies with beans and salsa)

LOW CARB LUNCH RECIPES

Grilled Chicken and Avocado Salad

Serves: 2

Cooking Time: 15 minutes

Ingredients:

- 6 ounces chicken breast (protein; for vegetarian, substitute with grilled tofu)
- 1 medium avocado, sliced (healthy fats, low carb)
- 2 cups mixed greens (fiber and vitamins; for leafy green sensitivities, substitute with arugula or spinach)
- 1/2 cup cherry tomatoes, halved (low carb, vitamin C; for nightshade intolerance, use sliced radishes)
- 1/2 cup cucumber, sliced (hydration, low carb)
- 2 tablespoons olive oil (healthy fats, for dressing)
- 1 tablespoon lemon juice (vitamin C, for dressing)
- Salt and pepper, to taste

Instructions:

- Preheat the grill to medium-high heat. Season the chicken breast (or tofu) with salt and pepper, and grill until fully cooked, about 6-7 minutes per side for

chicken or 3-4 minutes per side for tofu, until nicely charred and cooked through.
- While the chicken is grilling, prepare the salad by combining the mixed greens, cherry tomatoes (or radishes), cucumber, and avocado slices in a large salad bowl.
- In a small bowl, whisk together the olive oil and lemon juice, then season with salt and pepper to taste. This will be your dressing.
- Once the chicken (or tofu) is cooked and slightly cooled, slice it and add it to the salad.
- Drizzle the dressing over the salad and toss gently to combine everything.
- Serve the salad immediately, enjoying the blend of flavors and textures.

Note: Benefits of the Recipe

- Chicken breast offers a lean, high-quality protein source, essential for muscle maintenance, particularly beneficial for women over 50 and 60 to combat age-related muscle loss.
- Avocados provide heart-healthy monounsaturated fats, contributing to maintaining healthy cholesterol levels.

- The variety of mixed greens and vegetables delivers essential nutrients, supporting overall health, digestion, and offering anti-inflammatory benefits.

Nutritional Information (per serving):

- Calories: Approximately 400 kcal
- Protein: 35 g
- Total Fat: 25 g
- Saturated Fat: 4 g
- Carbohydrates: 12 g
- Dietary Fiber: 7 g
- Sugars: 2 g
- Sodium: 200 mg (varies with added salt)

Salmon and Asparagus Bundles

Serves: 2

Cooking Time: 20 minutes

Ingredients:

- 4 ounces salmon fillets (omega-3 fatty acids; for vegetarians, substitute with a large portobello mushroom cap)
- 6 asparagus spears (fiber, vitamins A, C, and E; for sensitivity, substitute with green beans)
- 1 tablespoon olive oil (healthy fats)
- 4 lemon slices (vitamin C)
- Dill, to taste (flavor)
- Salt and pepper, to taste

Instructions:

- Preheat the oven to 400°F (200°C) or prepare a grill for medium heat.
- Lay out two pieces of foil large enough to wrap the salmon and asparagus. Place the salmon in the center of each piece of foil.

- Arrange three asparagus spears (or green beans) alongside each salmon fillet. Drizzle with olive oil and season with salt, pepper, and dill.
- Place two lemon slices on top of each salmon.
- Wrap the foil around the salmon and asparagus, sealing the edges to form a bundle.
- Bake in the oven for 15-20 minutes or grill for 10-12 minutes, until the salmon is cooked through and the asparagus is tender.
- Carefully open the foil packets (watch for steam), and serve immediately.

Note: Benefits of the Recipe

- Salmon is an excellent source of omega-3 fatty acids, crucial for cardiovascular health and cognitive function.
- Asparagus provides a wealth of nutrients including fiber, folate, and vitamins A, C, and E, supporting heart health and offering antioxidant properties.
- Olive oil contributes beneficial antioxidants and monounsaturated fats, supporting heart health and reducing inflammation.

Nutritional Information (per serving):

- Calories: Approximately 300 kcal
- Protein: 23 g
- Total Fat: 20 g
- Saturated Fat: 3 g
- Carbohydrates: 5 g
- Dietary Fiber: 2 g
- Sugars: 2 g
- Sodium: 100 mg (varies with added salt)

Beef and Broccoli Stir-Fry

Serves: 2

Cooking Time: 20 minutes

Ingredients:

- 6 ounces lean beef slices (protein; for a vegetarian alternative, substitute with sliced tempeh)
- 1 cup broccoli florets (fiber, vitamins C and K; for sensitivity, substitute with bell peppers)
- 2 tablespoons soy sauce (flavor; for soy intolerance, substitute with coconut aminos)
- 1 teaspoon minced ginger (digestive aid)
- 1 clove minced garlic (antimicrobial; for intolerance, omit or use garlic-infused oil)
- 1 tablespoon olive oil (for stir-frying)
- 1 teaspoon sesame seeds (for garnish, optional)

Instructions:

- Heat the olive oil in a large skillet or wok over medium-high heat.
- Add the lean beef slices (or tempeh) and stir-fry until browned and nearly cooked through, about 3-4 minutes.

- Add the broccoli florets (or bell peppers), ginger, and garlic (or garlic-infused oil) to the skillet. Continue to stir-fry for another 5-7 minutes, or until the vegetables are tender and the beef is fully cooked.
- Stir in the soy sauce (or coconut aminos) and cook for an additional minute, allowing the flavors to meld.
- Serve the stir-fry hot, garnished with sesame seeds if desired.

Note: Benefits of the Recipe

- Lean beef provides a valuable source of protein and iron, supporting muscle maintenance and preventing anemia.
- Broccoli is rich in vitamins and minerals, aiding in detoxification and offering antioxidant protection.
- Ginger and garlic have health-promoting properties, including aiding digestion and providing anti-inflammatory benefits.

Nutritional Information (per serving):

- Calories: Approximately 300 kcal
- Protein: 26 g
- Total Fat: 15 g
- Saturated Fat: 3.5 g

- Carbohydrates: 10 g
- Dietary Fiber: 3 g
- Sugars: 2 g
- Sodium: 600 mg (varies with soy sauce and salt)

Turkey Lettuce Wraps

Serves: 2

Cooking Time: 15 minutes

Ingredients:

- 6 ounces ground turkey (lean protein; for vegetarian, substitute with crumbled tempeh)
- 4 large romaine lettuce leaves (low carb, hydration; for those with latex-fruit syndrome, substitute with kale leaves)
- 1 medium avocado, diced (healthy fats, low carb)
- 1/2 cup halved cherry tomatoes (low carb, vitamin C; for nightshade intolerance, substitute with diced red bell pepper)
- 1/4 cup finely chopped red onion (flavor; for those sensitive to alliums, substitute with thinly sliced radishes)
- 2 tablespoons chopped cilantro (flavor; for those who dislike cilantro, substitute with parsley)

- 2 tablespoons lime juice (vitamin C and flavor)
- 1 tablespoon olive oil (for cooking turkey)
- Salt and pepper, to taste

Instructions:

- Heat the olive oil in a skillet over medium heat. Add the ground turkey (or crumbled tempeh) and cook until browned and fully cooked through, breaking it into small pieces as it cooks. Season with salt and pepper.
- While the turkey is cooking, prepare the lettuce leaves (or kale leaves) by washing and drying them. Set aside for wrapping.
- In a small bowl, combine the diced avocado, halved cherry tomatoes (or diced red bell pepper), finely chopped red onion (or thinly sliced radishes), and chopped cilantro (or parsley). Squeeze the lime juice over the mixture and toss gently to combine.
- Once the turkey is cooked, remove from heat. Allow it to cool slightly before assembling the wraps.
- Place a generous spoonful of the turkey mixture onto the center of each lettuce leaf. Top with the avocado mixture.

- Fold the sides of the lettuce over the filling and roll up to enclose. Serve immediately.

Note: Benefits of the Recipe

- Ground turkey provides a lean source of protein, supporting muscle maintenance and growth, vital for combating sarcopenia in older adults.
- Avocado offers heart-healthy monounsaturated fats and fiber, promoting cardiovascular health and digestion.
- The combination of romaine lettuce and other vegetables delivers essential nutrients with minimal carbohydrate content, perfect for a low carb dietary approach.

Nutritional Information (per serving):

- Calories: Approximately 300 kcal
- Protein: 25 g
- Total Fat: 18 g
- Saturated Fat: 3 g
- Carbohydrates: 10 g
- Dietary Fiber: 6 g
- Sugars: 2 g
- Sodium: 200 mg (varies with added salt)

Shrimp and Spinach Salad

Serves: 2

Cooking Time: 10 minutes

Ingredients:

- 6 ounces shrimp (protein and omega-3 fatty acids; for shellfish allergy, substitute with grilled chicken breast)
- 2 cups spinach leaves (low carb, high in iron and vitamins A and C; for oxalate sensitivity, substitute with Swiss chard)
- 1/2 cup sliced cucumber (hydration, low carb)
- 1/4 cup crumbled feta cheese (calcium; for dairy intolerance, substitute with diced avocado)
- 2 tablespoons chopped walnuts (omega-3 fatty acids; for nut allergies, substitute with sunflower seeds)
- 2 tablespoons olive oil (healthy fats)
- 1 tablespoon balsamic vinegar (flavor; for low tolerance, use lemon juice)
- Salt and pepper, to taste

Instructions:

- If the shrimp isn't already cooked, boil or grill it until pink and opaque, then set aside to cool. If using chicken, grill until fully cooked and slice thinly.
- In a large salad bowl, combine the spinach leaves (or Swiss chard), sliced cucumber, crumbled feta cheese (or diced avocado), and chopped walnuts (or sunflower seeds).
- In a small bowl, whisk together the olive oil and balsamic vinegar (or lemon juice) to create the dressing. Season with salt and pepper.
- Add the cooled shrimp (or chicken) to the salad bowl. Drizzle the dressing over the salad and toss gently to combine.
- Serve the salad immediately, ensuring a mix of flavors and textures in each serving.

Note: Benefits of the Recipe

- Shrimp provides a lean source of protein and essential omega-3 fatty acids, aiding in weight management and muscle maintenance.
- Spinach offers a wealth of vitamins and minerals, supporting iron levels and overall nutritional health.

- The inclusion of olive oil and walnuts (or sunflower seeds) introduces healthy fats, beneficial for heart and cognitive function.

Nutritional Information (per serving):

- Calories: Approximately 350 kcal
- Protein: 25 g
- Total Fat: 22 g
- Saturated Fat: 4 g
- Carbohydrates: 8 g
- Dietary Fiber: 3 g
- Sugars: 2 g
- Sodium: 300 mg (varies with shrimp and added salt)

CONGRATULATIONS ON COMPLETING CHAPTER 3 OF OUR CARB CYCLING GUIDE

We sincerely hope that the lunch for the high carb and low carb recipes provided have not only tantalized your taste buds but also supported you in your journey towards managing carb intake effectively.

Each recipe within our guide has been meticulously designed to align with carb cycling principles, ensuring that you can enjoy your meals without concern for disrupting your dietary goals. Embracing these recipes signifies a proactive step in enhancing your overall health and well-being.

As we eagerly anticipate introducing you to an array of snacks and appetizer options in Chapter 4, we pause to seek your valued feedback.

Your insights and honest review of the breakfast recipes are crucial for us. They enable us to refine our approach, ensuring that we meet your expectations and assist others in navigating their carb cycling journey with greater confidence.

Thank you for contributing to our community's growth and for your commitment to exploring the carb cycling lifestyle. We are excited to guide you through the forthcoming chapter, where delicious, carb-conscious lunch recipes await. Your involvement is key to our collective success, and we look forward to hearing from you.

CHAPTER 4

HIGH CARB SNACKS AND APPETIZER

Fruit and Oat Energy Balls

Serves: 12 balls

Cooking Time: 10 minutes + chilling

- **Ingredients:**
- 1 cup rolled oats (high carb, fiber; for gluten intolerance, ensure gluten-free oats)
- 1/2 cup pitted and chopped Medjool dates (natural sweetness, high carb; for sensitivity, substitute with dried apricots)
- 1 large banana, mashed (natural sweetness, high carb)
- 2 tablespoons chia seeds (fiber and omega-3s; for intolerance, substitute with ground flaxseeds)
- 1 teaspoon cinnamon (flavor)
- 1/4 cup unsweetened shredded coconut (for coating; for coconut allergies, use crushed almonds or leave plain)

Instructions:

- In a large bowl, combine the rolled oats, chopped dates (or apricots), mashed banana, chia seeds (or ground flaxseeds), and cinnamon. Mix until well combined. The mixture should be sticky and hold together when pressed.
- Using your hands, form the mixture into small balls, about the size of a walnut.
- Place the shredded coconut (or crushed almonds) in a shallow dish. Roll each ball in the coconut to coat thoroughly.
- Place the energy balls on a baking sheet or plate lined with parchment paper. Refrigerate for at least 30 minutes to set.
- Enjoy these energy balls as a quick snack or energy boost. Store any leftovers in an airtight container in the refrigerator for up to a week.

Note: Benefits of the Recipe

- Rolled oats provide complex carbohydrates and fiber, promoting steady blood sugar levels and heart health.
- Medjool dates and bananas offer natural sugars for energy, along with potassium and dietary fiber for digestion and heart health.

- Chia seeds contribute omega-3 fatty acids, essential for brain health and reducing inflammation.

Nutritional Information (per ball):

- Calories: Approximately 100 kcal
- Protein: 2 g
- Total Fat: 3 g
- Saturated Fat: 1 g
- Carbohydrates: 18 g
- Dietary Fiber: 3 g
- Sugars: 8 g
- Sodium: LOW

Sweet Potato Hummus with Whole Wheat Pita

Serves: 4

Cooking Time: 15 minutes (excluding sweet potato cooking time)

Ingredients:

- 1 cup cooked and mashed sweet potatoes (high in complex carbs and vitamin A; for sensitivity, substitute with butternut squash)
- 1 cup cooked chickpeas (fiber and protein; for legume intolerance, substitute with white beans)
- 2 tablespoons tahini (sesame seed paste; for allergy, substitute with almond butter)
- 2 tablespoons lemon juice (vitamin C)
- 1 clove minced garlic (flavor; for intolerance, omit or use asafoetida)
- 1 teaspoon cumin (flavor)
- 2 whole wheat pita breads, cut into wedges (high carb; for gluten intolerance, use gluten-free pita or carrot sticks)

Instructions:

- In a food processor, combine the cooked sweet potatoes (or butternut squash), chickpeas (or white beans), tahini (or almond butter), lemon juice, garlic (or asafoetida), and cumin. Blend until smooth.
- If the hummus is too thick, you can add a little water or olive oil to reach your desired consistency. Season with salt and pepper to taste.
- Serve the sweet potato hummus with whole wheat pita wedges (or gluten-free pita/carrot sticks) for dipping.
- Enjoy this nutritious and satisfying snack or appetizer.

Note: Benefits of the Recipe

- Sweet potatoes and chickpeas provide a rich source of complex carbohydrates, fiber, and vitamins, supporting energy levels and muscle health.
- Tahini and lemon juice add healthy fats and vitamin C, enhancing flavor and nutritional value.

Nutritional Information (per serving):

- Calories: Approximately 300 kcal
- Protein: 9 g
- Total Fat: 8 g

- Saturated Fat: 1 g
- Carbohydrates: 50 g
- Dietary Fiber: 8 g
- Sugars: 7 g
- Sodium: Moderate

High Carb Quinoa Fruit Salad

Serves: 4

Cooking Time: 10 minutes (excluding quinoa cooking time)

Ingredients:

- 1 cup cooked quinoa (high carb, complete protein; for sensitivity, substitute with couscous)
- 1 cup mixed fresh berries (antioxidants, vitamins; for sensitivities, use diced mango or peaches)
- 1 medium apple, diced (fiber, natural sweetness)
- 2 tablespoons honey (natural sweetener; for avoidance, substitute with maple syrup)
- 1 tablespoon lime juice (vitamin C and flavor)
- 2 tablespoons chopped mint leaves (flavor; if intolerant to mint, omit or substitute with basil)

Instructions:

- In a large bowl, combine the cooked quinoa, mixed berries (or mango/peaches), and diced apple.
- In a small bowl, whisk together the honey (or maple syrup) and lime juice until well combined.

- Pour the honey-lime dressing over the quinoa and fruit mixture. Add the chopped mint (or basil) and gently toss to coat evenly.
- Chill the salad for at least 30 minutes before serving to allow the flavors to meld.
- Serve this refreshing and nutritious salad as a side dish or a light meal.

Note: Benefits of the Recipe

- Quinoa offers a high-carb, complete protein source, providing all essential amino acids for muscle repair and growth.
- Fresh fruits contribute vitamins, antioxidants, and dietary fiber, supporting overall health and preventing chronic diseases.
- Honey and lime juice provide natural sweetness and flavor, enhancing the salad's taste without processed sugars.

Nutritional Information (per serving):

- Calories: Approximately 250 kcal
- Protein: 6 g
- Total Fat: 2 g
- Saturated Fat: 0 g

- Carbohydrates: 52 g
- Dietary Fiber: 6 g
- Sugars: 25 g
- Sodium: Low

Baked Sweet Potato Fries with Greek Yogurt Dip

Serves: 4

Cooking Time: 30 minutes

Ingredients:

- 2 large sweet potatoes, cut into fries (high in complex carbs and vitamin A; for sensitivity, substitute with parsnips)
- 2 tablespoons olive oil (healthy fats)
- 1 teaspoon paprika (for flavor; if intolerant, substitute with dried herbs like thyme)
- 1/2 teaspoon salt (to taste)
- 1/2 cup Greek yogurt (protein; for dairy intolerance, substitute with coconut yogurt)
- 1 tablespoon lime juice (vitamin C)
- 1/2 teaspoon garlic powder (flavor; for garlic intolerance, omit or use a pinch of asafoetida powder)

- 2 tablespoons fresh cilantro, chopped (flavor; if intolerant to cilantro, substitute with parsley)

Instructions:

- Preheat your oven to 425°F (220°C). Line a baking sheet with parchment paper.
- Toss the sweet potato fries with olive oil, paprika (or dried herbs), and salt in a large bowl until evenly coated.
- Spread the fries in a single layer on the prepared baking sheet. Bake for 25-30 minutes, turning once halfway through, until crispy and golden brown.
- While the fries are baking, prepare the dip. In a small bowl, combine Greek yogurt (or coconut yogurt), lime juice, garlic powder (or asafoetida), and chopped cilantro (or parsley). Mix well and refrigerate until ready to serve.
- Serve the baked sweet potato fries hot with the Greek yogurt dip on the side.

Note: Benefits of the Recipe

- Sweet potatoes provide a nutritious source of carbohydrates and fiber, supporting steady blood

sugar levels and contributing to immune function and eye health with their beta-carotene content.
- Greek yogurt offers a good source of protein and probiotics, enhancing digestive health and bone density, which are crucial for women over 50 and 60.

Nutritional Information (per serving):

- Calories: Approximately 200 kcal
- Protein: 5 g
- Total Fat: 7 g
- Saturated Fat: 1 g
- Carbohydrates: 30 g
- Dietary Fiber: 4 g
- Sugars: 7 g
- Sodium: 300 mg (varies with added salt)

Quinoa and Black Bean Stuffed Peppers

Serves: 4

Cooking Time: 45 minutes

Ingredients:

- 1 cup cooked quinoa (high carb, complete protein; for sensitivity, substitute with bulgur wheat)
- 1 cup cooked black beans (fiber and protein; for intolerance, substitute with chopped mushrooms)
- 4 medium bell peppers (vitamin C and potassium; for nightshade intolerance, substitute with hollowed-out zucchini)
- 1/2 cup corn kernels (high carb, fiber; for intolerance, substitute with peas)
- 1/4 cup finely diced onion (flavor; for sensitivity, substitute with fennel)
- 1 teaspoon cumin (flavor)
- 2 tablespoons chopped cilantro (flavor; if intolerant to cilantro, substitute with parsley)
- 1 tablespoon lime juice (vitamin C and flavor)

Instructions:

- Preheat the oven to 375°F (190°C). Cut the tops off the bell peppers (or zucchini) and remove the seeds. Set aside.
- In a large bowl, mix the cooked quinoa, black beans (or mushrooms), corn kernels (or peas), diced onion (or fennel), cumin, cilantro (or parsley), and lime juice. Season with salt and pepper to taste.
- Stuff the mixture evenly into the bell peppers (or hollowed-out zucchini). Place the stuffed peppers in a baking dish.
- Bake in the preheated oven for about 30 minutes, or until the peppers are tender and the filling is heated through.
- Serve the stuffed peppers warm, with additional lime wedges on the side if desired.

Note: Benefits of the Recipe

- Quinoa provides a high-carbohydrate and complete protein source, essential for maintaining muscle mass and energy levels, particularly beneficial for older adults.
- Black beans and bell peppers offer a combination of fiber, protein, and vitamins A and C, supporting

cardiovascular health, stable blood sugar levels, and immune function.

Nutritional Information (per serving):

- Calories: Approximately 250 kcal
- Protein: 10 g
- Total Fat: 2 g
- Saturated Fat: 0 g
- Carbohydrates: 50 g
- Dietary Fiber: 10 g
- Sugars: 5 g
- Sodium: 200 mg (varies with added salt)

LOW CARB SNACKS AND APPETIZER

Avocado Cucumber Rolls

Serves: 2

Cooking Time: 10 minutes

Ingredients:

- 1 large cucumber, thinly sliced (hydration and vitamins, low carb; for sensitivity, substitute with zucchini strips)
- 1 medium avocado, mashed (healthy fats, low carb)
- 1 tablespoon lime juice (vitamin C)
- 4 ounces smoked salmon (protein and omega-3 fatty acids; for vegetarians, substitute with thin slices of tofu)
- 1 tablespoon fresh dill, chopped (flavor; if intolerant, substitute with fresh chives)
- Salt and pepper, to taste

Instructions:

- Use a vegetable peeler or mandoline slicer to cut long, thin slices of cucumber (or zucchini).
- In a small bowl, mix the mashed avocado with lime juice, chopped dill (or chives), and season with salt and pepper to taste.
- Lay out the cucumber slices and spread a thin layer of the avocado mixture onto each slice.
- Place a small piece of smoked salmon (or tofu) on one end of each cucumber slice.
- Carefully roll up the cucumber slices around the salmon/tofu, securing with a toothpick if necessary.
- Serve immediately as a fresh and nutritious appetizer or snack.

Note: Benefits of the Recipe

- Cucumbers and avocados offer a hydrating and heart-healthy combination, providing essential vitamins and monounsaturated fats.
- Smoked salmon enriches the dish with omega-3 fatty acids, important for brain health and reducing inflammation, making it a great choice for overall wellness.

Nutritional Information (per serving):

- Calories: Approximately 300 kcal
- Protein: 14 g
- Total Fat: 22 g
- Saturated Fat: 3 g
- Carbohydrates: 12 g
- Dietary Fiber: 7 g
- Sugars: 3 g
- Sodium: 600 mg (varies with smoked salmon and added salt)

Stuffed Mini Bell Peppers

Serves: 4

Cooking Time: 20 minutes

Ingredients:

- 8 mini bell peppers, halved and seeded (vitamin C and A, low carb; for nightshade intolerance, substitute with celery sticks)
- 4 ounces cream cheese (fat; for dairy intolerance, substitute with almond or coconut cream cheese)
- 1/4 cup shredded cheddar cheese (calcium; for dairy intolerance, use dairy-free cheese)
- 2 tablespoons chopped green onions (flavor; for sensitivity, substitute with dried herbs)
- 1/2 teaspoon garlic powder (flavor; for intolerance, omit or use asafoetida)
- Salt and pepper, to taste

Instructions:

- Preheat the oven to 375°F (190°C). Arrange the halved mini bell peppers on a baking sheet.
- In a bowl, mix together the cream cheese (or non-dairy alternative), shredded cheddar cheese (or non-

dairy cheese), chopped green onions (or dried herbs), garlic powder (or asafoetida), and season with salt and pepper.
- Fill each bell pepper half with the cheese mixture, pressing gently to ensure it's packed well.
- Bake in the preheated oven for 10-15 minutes, or until the peppers are tender and the cheese is bubbly.
- Serve warm as a delicious and colorful appetizer or side dish.

Note: Benefits of the Recipe

- Mini bell peppers provide a nutrient-rich base, offering essential vitamins for immune function and eye health.
- The combination of cheeses (or dairy-free alternatives) adds creaminess and flavor, along with calcium for bone health.

Nutritional Information (per serving):

- Calories: Approximately 200 kcal
- Protein: 6 g
- Total Fat: 15 g
- Saturated Fat: 8 g
- Carbohydrates: 8 g

- Dietary Fiber: 2 g
- Sugars: 4 g
- Sodium: 300 mg (varies with cheese and added salt)

Zucchini Chips with Herbed Yogurt Dip

Serves: 4

Cooking Time: 25 minutes

Ingredients:

- 2 large zucchini, sliced thinly (fiber and vitamins, low carb; for sensitivity, substitute with sliced radishes)
- 1 tablespoon olive oil (healthy fats)
- 1/2 teaspoon salt (to taste)
- 1/2 cup Greek yogurt (protein; for dairy intolerance, substitute with coconut yogurt)
- 1 teaspoon lemon zest (flavor and vitamins)
- 2 tablespoons finely chopped fresh herbs (dill, parsley, or chives, depending on tolerance)
- 1/2 teaspoon garlic powder (flavor; for intolerance, omit)

Instructions:

- Preheat your oven to 425°F (220°C). Line a baking sheet with parchment paper.
- Toss the thinly sliced zucchini (or radishes) with olive oil and salt, then spread in a single layer on the baking sheet.
- Bake for 15-20 minutes, turning halfway through, until crispy and golden.
- While the zucchini chips are baking, prepare the dip. Mix the Greek yogurt (or coconut yogurt) with lemon zest, chopped herbs, and garlic powder (if using) in a small bowl.
- Serve the crispy zucchini chips with the herbed yogurt dip on the side.

Note: Benefits of the Recipe

- Zucchini offers a low-carb option packed with vitamins and fiber, promoting digestion and skin health.
- The herbed yogurt dip provides a protein boost and probiotics for gut health, along with the added flavor from fresh herbs and lemon zest.

Nutritional Information (per serving):

- Calories: Approximately 100 kcal
- Protein: 4 g
- Total Fat: 6 g
- Saturated Fat: 1 g
- Carbohydrates: 8 g
- Dietary Fiber: 2 g
- Sugars: 4 g
- Sodium: 300 mg (varies with added salt)

Cauliflower Hummus with Vegetable Sticks

Serves: 4

Cooking Time: 15 minutes (excluding steaming time)

Ingredients:

- 2 cups steamed and cooled cauliflower (low carb, high in vitamins C and K; for those sensitive to cruciferous vegetables, substitute with steamed zucchini)
- 2 tablespoons tahini (sesame paste; for sesame allergies, substitute with almond butter)
- 2 tablespoons olive oil (healthy fats)
- 2 tablespoons lemon juice (vitamin C)
- 1 clove minced garlic (antioxidant; for garlic intolerance, omit or use a pinch of asafoetida powder)
- 1 teaspoon cumin (flavor; if intolerant, substitute with paprika)
- 1/2 teaspoon salt (to taste)
- Assorted vegetable sticks (carrots, celery, cucumber; for specific intolerances, choose tolerated vegetables) for serving

Instructions:

- In a food processor, combine the steamed and cooled cauliflower (or zucchini), tahini (or almond butter), olive oil, lemon juice, garlic (or asafoetida), cumin (or paprika), and salt. Blend until smooth and creamy. Adjust the seasoning to taste.
- Transfer the hummus to a serving bowl. Chill in the refrigerator for at least 1 hour to allow the flavors to meld.
- Serve the cauliflower hummus with an assortment of vegetable sticks such as carrots, celery, and cucumber, or any other tolerated vegetables.
- Enjoy this healthy and nutritious alternative to traditional hummus as a snack or appetizer.

Note: Benefits of the Recipe

- Cauliflower serves as a low-carb alternative to chickpeas, offering essential vitamins for immune support and bone health.
- Olive oil and tahini contribute healthy fats and essential minerals, promoting heart health and aiding in calcium and zinc intake.

Nutritional Information (per serving):

- Calories: Approximately 150 kcal
- Protein: 3 g
- Total Fat: 12 g
- Saturated Fat: 2 g
- Carbohydrates: 8 g
- Dietary Fiber: 3 g
- Sugars: 3 g
- Sodium: 300 mg (varies with added salt)

Avocado and Salmon Salad Cups

Serves: 4

Cooking Time: 10 minutes

Ingredients:

- 4 ounces smoked salmon (omega-3 fatty acids; for vegetarians, substitute with extra avocado)
- 1 large avocado, diced (healthy fats, low carb)
- 1/2 cup diced cucumber (hydration, low carb)
- 8 endive leaves (serving cups, low carb; for intolerance, use romaine lettuce)
- 1 tablespoon chopped dill (flavor; if intolerant, substitute with parsley)
- 1 tablespoon lemon juice (vitamin C)
- Salt and pepper, to taste

Instructions:

- In a medium bowl, combine the diced avocado, diced cucumber, and chopped dill (or parsley). Squeeze the lemon juice over the mixture and gently toss to combine. Season with salt and pepper to taste.
- Arrange the endive leaves (or romaine lettuce leaves) on a serving platter.

- Divide the smoked salmon (or additional avocado for vegetarians) among the endive cups.
- Top the salmon with the avocado and cucumber mixture, distributing it evenly among the cups.
- Serve immediately as a refreshing and nutritious appetizer or light meal, perfect for any occasion.

Note: Benefits of the Recipe

- Smoked salmon and avocado provide a rich source of omega-3 fatty acids and monounsaturated fats, supporting heart and cognitive function.
- The combination of endive, cucumber, and lemon juice adds hydration and essential nutrients with minimal carbohydrates, making it a healthy and satisfying option.

Nutritional Information (per serving):

- Calories: Approximately 200 kcal
- Protein: 10 g
- Total Fat: 15 g
- Saturated Fat: 2.5 g
- Carbohydrates: 8 g
- Dietary Fiber: 5 g
- Sugars: 1 g

CONGRATULATIONS ON COMPLETING CHAPTER 4 OF OUR CARB CYCLING GUIDE

We sincerely hope that the SNACKS AND APPETIZER for the high carb and low carb recipes provided have not only tantalized your taste buds but also supported you in your journey towards managing carb intake effectively.

Each recipe within our guide has been meticulously designed to align with carb cycling principles, ensuring that you can enjoy your meals without concern for disrupting your dietary goals. Embracing these recipes signifies a proactive step in enhancing your overall health and well-being.

As we eagerly anticipate introducing you to an array of dinner options in Chapter5, we pause to seek your valued feedback.

Your insights and honest review of the breakfast recipes are crucial for us. They enable us to refine our approach, ensuring that we meet your expectations and assist others in navigating their carb cycling journey with greater confidence.

Thank you for contributing to our community's growth and for your commitment to exploring the carb cycling lifestyle. We are excited to guide you through the forthcoming chapter, where delicious, carb-conscious lunch recipes await. Your involvement is key to our collective success, and we look forward to hearing from you.

CHAPTER 5

HIGH CARB DINNER RECIPES

Gnocchi with Tomato Sauce and Fresh Basil

Serves: 4

Cooking Time: 30 minutes

Ingredients:

- 500g gnocchi (high carb, provides energy)
- 2 cups tomato sauce (rich in lycopene, antioxidants)
- A handful of fresh basil (anti-inflammatory properties)
- 50g Parmesan cheese (can substitute with nutritional yeast for dairy intolerance)
- 1 tbsp olive oil (healthy fats)

Instructions:

- Bring a large pot of salted water to a boil. Add the gnocchi and cook according to the package instructions until they float to the top, then drain.
- In a large skillet, heat the olive oil over medium heat. Add the tomato sauce and warm through.

- Add the cooked gnocchi to the skillet with the tomato sauce. Stir gently to coat the gnocchi in the sauce.
- Serve the gnocchi topped with freshly grated Parmesan cheese (or nutritional yeast) and a generous sprinkle of fresh basil leaves.
- Enjoy this comforting dish, perfect for refueling on high carb days.

Note: Benefits of the Recipe

- Gnocchi provides a satisfying source of carbohydrates, ideal for energy replenishment.
- Tomato sauce and basil contribute antioxidants and anti-inflammatory compounds, supporting overall health.

Nutritional Information (per serving):

- Calories: Approximately 350 kcal
- Protein: 10 g
- Total Fat: 7 g
- Saturated Fat: 2 g
- Carbohydrates: 60 g
- Dietary Fiber: 4 g
- Sugars: 4 g

- Sodium: Moderate (varies with tomato sauce and added salt)

Seafood Alfredo Pasta

Serves: 4

Cooking Time: 30 minutes

Ingredients:

- 400g pasta (high carb, energy source)
- 500g mixed seafood (lean protein, omega-3 fatty acids)
- 1 cup Alfredo sauce (can substitute with a cashew-based sauce for lactose intolerance)
- 2 cloves garlic, minced
- 2 tbsp olive oil
- Parsley for garnish (optional)

Instructions:

- Cook the pasta according to package instructions until al dente. Drain and set aside.
- In a large skillet, heat the olive oil over medium heat. Add the minced garlic and sauté until fragrant.

- Add the mixed seafood to the skillet and cook until just done, about 5-7 minutes, depending on the seafood used.
- Lower the heat and stir in the Alfredo sauce (or cashew-based sauce) until the seafood is coated and the sauce is heated through.
- Toss the cooked pasta with the seafood Alfredo mixture until well combined.
- Serve garnished with parsley, offering a rich and fulfilling meal packed with protein and healthy fats.

Note: Benefits of the Recipe

- Pasta serves as a significant source of energy, supporting endurance and recovery.
- Seafood provides high-quality protein and omega-3 fatty acids, important for muscle repair and heart health.

Nutritional Information (per serving):

- Calories: Approximately 600 kcal
- Protein: 35 g
- Total Fat: 20 g
- Saturated Fat: 5 g
- Carbohydrates: 75 g

- Dietary Fiber: 3 g
- Sugars: 3 g
- Sodium: High (varies with Alfredo sauce and added salt)

Eggplant Parmesan with Spaghetti

Serves: 4

Cooking Time: 1 hour

Ingredients:

- 2 medium eggplants, sliced (fiber, antioxidants)
- 400g spaghetti (high carb, energy source)
- 2 cups tomato sauce
- 200g mozzarella cheese (can substitute with a dairy-free alternative)
- 50g Parmesan cheese (or nutritional yeast)
- 2 tbsp olive oil

Instructions:

- Preheat the oven to 375°F (190°C). Arrange eggplant slices on a baking sheet, brush with olive oil, and season with salt. Bake until tender, about 20 minutes.
- Cook the spaghetti according to package instructions until al dente. Drain and set aside.

- In a baking dish, layer the baked eggplant slices, tomato sauce, and mozzarella cheese. Repeat until all ingredients are used, finishing with a layer of cheese.
- Bake in the preheated oven for 30 minutes, or until the cheese is bubbly and golden.
- Serve the eggplant Parmesan over the cooked spaghetti, garnished with Parmesan cheese (or nutritional yeast).

Note: Benefits of the Recipe

- Eggplant and spaghetti provide a hearty source of carbohydrates and fiber, enhancing digestive health and energy levels.
- Cheese adds calcium and protein, supporting bone health and muscle repair.

Nutritional Information (per serving):

- Calories: Approximately 550 kcal
- Protein: 25 g
- Total Fat: 20 g
- Saturated Fat: 8 g
- Carbohydrates: 75 g
- Dietary Fiber: 8 g
- Sugars: 10 g

- Sodium: High (varies with tomato sauce and added salt)

Korean BBQ Beef with Steamed Rice

Serves: 4

Cooking Time: 30 minutes

Ingredients:

- 500g beef slices (lean protein, iron source)
- 1 cup Korean BBQ sauce (can be made with gluten-free soy sauce for gluten intolerance)
- 2 cups steamed rice (high carb, primary energy source)
- 2 tbsp sesame oil (healthy fats, anti-inflammatory)
- A handful of green onions for garnish

Instructions:

- Marinate the beef slices in the Korean BBQ sauce for at least 30 minutes, or overnight in the refrigerator for deeper flavor.
- Heat a grill pan or skillet over medium-high heat. Add the sesame oil, and then cook the marinated beef slices for 2-3 minutes on each side, or until nicely charred and cooked to your preference.

- While the beef is cooking, steam the rice according to package instructions until fluffy.
- Serve the Korean BBQ beef over the steamed rice, garnished with chopped green onions.

Note: Benefits of the Recipe

- Provides a balanced meal with high-quality protein from beef, complex carbohydrates from rice, and healthy fats from sesame oil.
- Korean BBQ sauce and green onions add flavor and nutrients, including antioxidants and vitamins.

Nutritional Information (per serving):

- Calories: Approximately 500 kcal
- Protein: 30 g
- Total Fat: 15 g
- Saturated Fat: 4 g
- Carbohydrates: 60 g
- Dietary Fiber: 1 g
- Sugars: 10 g (varies with BBQ sauce)
- Sodium: High (varies with BBQ sauce and added salt)

Chicken Tikka Masala with Basmati Rice

Serves: 4

Cooking Time: 45 minutes

Ingredients:

- 500g chicken breast, cut into chunks (lean protein source, helps in muscle maintenance)
- 200g Greek yogurt (can substitute with lactose-free yogurt if intolerant)
- 3 tbsp tikka masala paste (spices can boost metabolism)
- 2 cups basmati rice (high carb, replenishes glycogen stores)
- 400g can canned tomatoes (rich in antioxidants)
- 2 tbsp olive oil (healthy fats, supports cardiovascular health)
- Cilantro for garnish (optional)

Instructions:

- In a bowl, combine the Greek yogurt and tikka masala paste. Add the chicken chunks and marinate for at least 30 minutes, preferably overnight in the fridge.

- Preheat the oven to 400°F (200°C). Place the marinated chicken on a baking tray and cook for 20-25 minutes, or until fully cooked.
- While the chicken is cooking, rinse the basmati rice until the water runs clear. Bring a pot of water to boil, add the rice, and cook according to package instructions until fluffy.
- Heat the olive oil in a skillet over medium heat. Add the canned tomatoes and let simmer for 10 minutes. Add the cooked chicken to the tomato sauce and mix well.
- Serve the chicken tikka masala over the cooked basmati rice, garnished with cilantro if desired.

Note: Benefits of the Recipe

- Provides a balanced meal with lean protein from chicken, complex carbohydrates from rice, and healthy fats from olive oil.
- Spices in tikka masala and the antioxidants from tomatoes contribute to boosting metabolism and supporting heart health.

Nutritional Information (per serving):

- Calories: Approximately 600 kcal
- Protein: 40 g
- Total Fat: 15 g
- Saturated Fat: 3 g
- Carbohydrates: 80 g
- Dietary Fiber: 2 g
- Sugars: 5 g
- Sodium: Moderate (varies with tikka masala paste and added salt)

LOW CARB DINNER RECIPES

Grilled Lemon-Herb Chicken and Zucchini

Serves: 4

Cooking Time: 20 minutes

Ingredients:

- 4 medium chicken breasts (lean protein; for vegetarian, substitute with portobello mushrooms)
- 2 large zucchini, sliced lengthwise (low carb, high in vitamins; for sensitivity, substitute with asparagus)
- 2 tablespoons olive oil (healthy fats)
- 2 tablespoons lemon juice (vitamin C)
- 2 cloves minced garlic (immune support; for intolerance, substitute with a pinch of asafoetida powder)
- 1 teaspoon each, chopped rosemary and thyme (antioxidants; if intolerant, substitute with oregano)
- Salt and pepper, to taste

Instructions:

- Preheat your grill to medium-high heat.

- In a small bowl, whisk together the olive oil, lemon juice, minced garlic (or asafoetida), rosemary, thyme (or oregano), salt, and pepper.
- Brush the chicken breasts (or portobello mushrooms) and zucchini slices with the lemon-herb mixture.
- Place the chicken (or mushrooms) and zucchini on the grill. Cook the chicken for about 6-7 minutes per side, or until fully cooked through. Grill the zucchini for about 3-4 minutes per side, or until tender and grill marks appear.
- Serve the grilled chicken (or mushrooms) and zucchini hot, garnished with additional herbs or lemon wedges if desired.

Note: Benefits of the Recipe

- Chicken and zucchini provide a low-carb, high-protein meal rich in vitamins and minerals, supporting muscle mass, eye health, and digestive health.
- Olive oil contributes heart-healthy fats, aiding in cardiovascular health and inflammation management.

Nutritional Information (per serving):

- Calories: Approximately 250 kcal
- Protein: 26 g

- Total Fat: 12 g
- Saturated Fat: 2 g
- Carbohydrates: 6 g
- Dietary Fiber: 2 g
- Sugars: 3 g
- Sodium: 200 mg (varies with added salt)

Beef and Mushroom Lettuce Wraps

Serves: 4

Cooking Time: 20 minutes

Ingredients:

- 1 pound lean ground beef (protein; for vegetarian, substitute with crumbled firm tofu)
- 1 cup chopped mushrooms (fiber and vitamins; for intolerance, substitute with diced bell peppers)
- 8 large lettuce leaves (serving wraps, low carb; for sensitivity, use kale leaves)
- 1 tablespoon avocado oil (healthy fats)
- 2 tablespoons chopped green onions (flavor; for allium intolerance, omit or use chives)
- 1 tablespoon grated ginger (digestive aid)
- 2 tablespoons soy sauce (umami flavor; for soy intolerance, use coconut aminos)
- 1 teaspoon sesame seeds for garnish (calcium; for allergies, omit)

Instructions:

- Heat avocado oil in a large skillet over medium heat. Add the ground beef (or tofu) and cook until browned, breaking it up with a spoon as it cooks.
- Add the chopped mushrooms (or bell peppers), green onions (or chives), and grated ginger to the skillet. Cook for an additional 5-7 minutes, until the vegetables are tender.
- Stir in the soy sauce (or coconut aminos) and cook for another minute, allowing the flavors to meld together.
- Spoon the beef (or tofu) mixture into the lettuce (or kale) leaves. Garnish with sesame seeds if using.
- Serve immediately, enjoying the flavorful and nutritious wraps as a low-carb, high-protein meal.

Note: Benefits of the Recipe

- Lean ground beef or tofu provides a solid protein base, supporting muscle health and energy levels.
- Mushrooms and lettuce contribute essential nutrients and fiber, promoting immune function and digestive health.

Nutritional Information (per serving):

- Calories: Approximately 300 kcal
- Protein: 25 g
- Total Fat: 18 g
- Saturated Fat: 5 g
- Carbohydrates: 8 g
- Dietary Fiber: 2 g
- Sugars: 3 g
- Sodium: 500 mg (varies with soy sauce and added salt)

Salmon and Avocado Salad

Serves: 4

Cooking Time: 15 minutes

Ingredients:

- 4 ounces per serving salmon fillets (omega-3 fatty acids; for vegetarians, substitute with sliced avocados for additional healthy fats)
- 2 cups mixed greens (low carb, high in fiber; for intolerance, use spinach)
- 1 large avocado, diced (healthy fats, low carb)
- 1/2 cup sliced cucumber (hydration, low carb)
- 2 tablespoons olive oil (for dressing)
- 2 tablespoons lemon juice (for dressing)
- 1 tablespoon chopped dill (flavor; if intolerant, substitute with parsley)
- Salt and pepper, to taste

Instructions:

- Grill or bake the salmon fillets until cooked through and flaky. Set aside to cool slightly.
- In a large salad bowl, combine the mixed greens, diced avocado, and sliced cucumber.

- In a small bowl, whisk together the olive oil, lemon juice, chopped dill (or parsley), salt, and pepper to create the dressing.
- Break the salmon into bite-sized pieces and add to the salad bowl. Drizzle the dressing over the salad and gently toss to combine.
- Serve the salad immediately, offering a nutrient-rich, low-carb meal with healthy fats and essential vitamins.

Note: Benefits of the Recipe

- Salmon and avocado provide omega-3 and monounsaturated fats, crucial for brain health, reducing inflammation, and supporting cardiovascular health.
- Mixed greens and cucumber add a high volume of low-calorie nutrition, enhancing hydration and providing dietary fiber.

Nutritional Information (per serving):

- Calories: Approximately 350 kcal
- Protein: 24 g
- Total Fat: 25 g
- Saturated Fat: 4 g

- Carbohydrates: 10 g
- Dietary Fiber: 7 g
- Sugars: 2 g
- Sodium: 200 mg (varies with added salt)

Herb-Crusted Pork Tenderloin with Roasted Asparagus

Serves: 4

Cooking Time: 40 minutes

Ingredients:

- 1 pound pork tenderloin (lean protein; for a vegetarian alternative, substitute with whole roasted cauliflower)
- 1 tablespoon each, chopped fresh rosemary and thyme (flavor, antioxidants; if intolerant, substitute with dried Italian seasoning)
- 2 tablespoons olive oil (healthy fats, low carb)
- 1 pound asparagus, ends trimmed (fiber, vitamins A, C, E; for sensitivity, substitute with green beans)
- 2 cloves minced garlic (immune support; for intolerance, use a pinch of asafoetida powder)
- Salt and pepper, to taste

Instructions:

- Preheat your oven to 400°F (200°C).

- Rub the pork tenderloin with 1 tablespoon of olive oil. Season with the chopped rosemary, thyme (or Italian seasoning), salt, and pepper. Place in a roasting pan.
- In a separate bowl, toss the asparagus (or green beans) with the remaining tablespoon of olive oil, minced garlic (or asafoetida), and a sprinkle of salt and pepper.
- Arrange the asparagus around the pork in the roasting pan.
- Roast in the preheated oven for 25-30 minutes, or until the pork reaches an internal temperature of 145°F (63°C) and the asparagus is tender.
- Let the pork rest for 5 minutes before slicing. Serve the herb-crusted pork tenderloin with the roasted asparagus on the side.

Note: Benefits of the Recipe

- Pork tenderloin and asparagus provide a nutrient-dense meal, high in protein, fiber, and essential vitamins, supporting muscle maintenance, heart health, and immune function.
- Olive oil adds healthy fats, enhancing flavor and nutrient absorption.

Nutritional Information (per serving):

- Calories: Approximately 300 kcal
- Protein: 30 g
- Total Fat: 15 g
- Saturated Fat: 3 g
- Carbohydrates: 8 g
- Dietary Fiber: 3 g
- Sugars: 2 g
- Sodium: 300 mg (varies with added salt)

Grilled Chicken Caesar Salad

Serves: 4

Cooking Time: 20 minutes

Ingredients:

- 2 medium chicken breasts, grilled and sliced (protein; for a vegetarian option, substitute with grilled tofu)
- 4 cups chopped romaine lettuce (low carb, hydration; for intolerance, substitute with kale)
- 1/4 cup shaved Parmesan cheese (calcium; for dairy intolerance, substitute with nutritional yeast)
- 3 tablespoons Caesar dressing (low carb; for a healthier option, use a mixture of Greek yogurt with lemon juice, minced anchovies, and garlic)
- 1/4 cup chopped almonds (healthy fats, protein; for nut allergies, substitute with sunflower seeds)
- Lemon wedges (vitamin C), to serve
- Salt and pepper, to taste

Instructions:

- In a large salad bowl, combine the chopped romaine lettuce (or kale) with the grilled and sliced chicken (or tofu).

- Add the shaved Parmesan cheese (or nutritional yeast) to the salad.
- Drizzle the Caesar dressing over the salad and toss well to coat all the ingredients evenly.
- Sprinkle the chopped almonds (or sunflower seeds) over the top of the salad.
- Serve the salad with lemon wedges on the side, allowing individuals to add extra vitamin C to their taste.
- Season with salt and pepper as needed, and enjoy this classic salad with a nutritious twist.

Note: Benefits of the Recipe

- Chicken (or tofu) and romaine lettuce provide a low-carb option packed with protein and essential nutrients, supporting muscle health and hydration.
- Parmesan cheese (or nutritional yeast) and almonds (or sunflower seeds) add flavor and texture, along with calcium and healthy fats.

Nutritional Information (per serving):

- Calories: Approximately 250 kcal
- Protein: 25 g
- Total Fat: 14 g

- Saturated Fat: 3 g
- Carbohydrates: 6 g
- Dietary Fiber: 2 g
- Sugars: 2 g
- Sodium: 400 mg (varies with dressing and added salt)

CHAPTER 6

7 DAYS DAILY MEAL PLAN

Monday: High-Carb + Strength Training

6:30 AM: Breakfast - Oatmeal with Mixed Berries and Nuts

9:00 AM: Workout - Full body strength training (60 minutes)

11:00 AM: Snack - Fruit and Oat Energy Balls

1:00 PM: Lunch - Sweet Potato Chickpea Salad

4:00 PM: Snack - Quinoa and Black Bean Stuffed Peppers

7:00 PM: Dinner - Gnocchi with Tomato Sauce and Fresh Basil

Tuesday: Low-Carb + Light Activity (Yoga or Walk)

7:00 AM: Breakfast - Avocado and Egg Breakfast Bowl

10:00 AM: Light Activity - Gentle yoga session or a 30-minute walk

12:00 PM: Lunch - Grilled Chicken and Avocado Salad

3:00 PM: Snack - Zucchini Chips with Herbed Yogurt Dip

6:00 PM: Dinner - Beef and Mushroom Lettuce Wraps

Wednesday: High-Carb + HIIT

6:30 AM: Breakfast - Banana Pancakes with Maple Syrup and Fresh Fruit

9:00 AM: Workout - High-Intensity Interval Training (HIIT) for 30 minutes

11:00 AM: Snack - Sweet Potato Hummus with Whole Wheat Pita

1:00 PM: Lunch - Pasta Primavera with Whole Wheat Pasta

4:00 PM: Snack - High Carb Quinoa Fruit Salad

7:00 PM: Dinner - Seafood Alfredo Pasta

Thursday: Low-Carb + Rest Day

7:00 AM: Breakfast - Mushroom and Spinach Frittata

Rest Day: Engage in gentle stretching or a leisurely walk if desired

12:00 PM: Lunch - Turkey Lettuce Wraps

3:00 PM: Snack - Cauliflower Hummus with Vegetable Sticks

6:00 PM: Dinner - Herb-Crusted Pork Tenderloin with Roasted Asparagus

Friday: High-Carb + Circuit Training

6:30 AM: Breakfast - Tropical Mango and Coconut Rice Pudding

9:00 AM: Workout - Circuit training (45 minutes)

11:00 AM: Snack - Baked Sweet Potato Fries with Greek Yogurt Dip

1:00 PM: Lunch - Mediterranean Quinoa Salad

4:00 PM: Snack - Fruit and Oat Energy Balls

7:00 PM: Dinner - Chicken Tikka Masala with Basmati Rice

Saturday: Low-Carb + Light Activity (Swimming or Cycling)

7:00 AM: Breakfast - Zucchini and Bell Pepper Mini Quiches

10:00 AM: Light Activity - 30 minutes of swimming or cycling

12:00 PM: Lunch - Salmon and Asparagus Bundles

3:00 PM: Snack - Avocado Cucumber Rolls

6:00 PM: Dinner - Grilled Lemon-Herb Chicken and Zucchini

Sunday: Low-Carb + Rest Day

8:00 AM: Breakfast - Cauliflower Hash Browns

Rest Day: Consider mindfulness activities like meditation or gentle yoga

12:00 PM: Lunch - Shrimp and Spinach Salad

3:00 PM: Snack - Stuffed Mini Bell Peppers

6:00 PM: Dinner - Grilled Chicken Caesar Salad

2 WEEKS MEAL PLANNER

AMOS JIMMY
DAILY MEAL PLANNER

DATE ————————   M T W T F S S

BREAKFAST

DINNER

LUNCH

NOTES

SNACKS

JIMMY'S CULINARY HAVEN

AMOS JIMMY
DAILY MEAL PLANNER

DATE: _____   M T W T F S S

BREAKFAST

DINNER

LUNCH

NOTES

SNACKS

JIMMY'S CULINARY HAVEN

Jimmy Asking For An Honest Review

I wanted to reach out and personally thank you for taking the time to explore the world of flavors and creations that I poured into those pages.

Your experience matters a lot to me, and I would be truly grateful if you could share your honest thoughts in a review. Whether it's a brief note or a detailed reflection, your feedback will not only help me grow as a creator but also guide fellow food enthusiasts in deciding if this cookbook is a culinary adventure they'd like to embark on.

Feel free to highlight your favorite recipes, share any challenges you conquered, or even suggest what you'd love to see more of in future editions. Your unique perspective adds a special spice to the whole mix!

Thank you again for being a part of this delicious journey. I can't wait to hear what you think!

Made in the USA
Las Vegas, NV
15 October 2024